The Automatic 6-Pack Workout

THE PREMIER WORKOUT GUIDE FOR GAINING LEAN MUSCLE, LOSING BELLY FAT, AND IMPROVING YOUR OVERALL HEALTH

John Andre

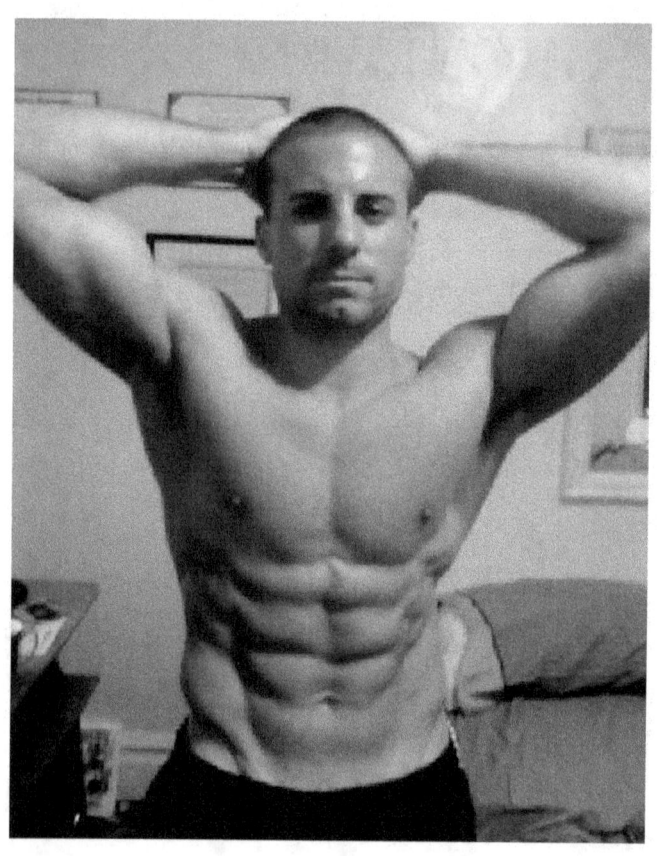

DISCLAIMER

The author, John Andre, strongly recommends that you consult with your physician before beginning any exercise program.

You need to be in good physical condition and able to participate in strenuous exercises.

John Andre is not a licensed physical trainer or medical care provider. He fully discloses that he has no expertise in diagnosing, examining, or treating medical conditions of any kind, or in determining the effect of any specific exercise on a medical condition.

You should understand that when participating in any exercise or exercise program, there is the possibility of physical injury. If you engage in this exercise or exercise program, you agree that you do so at your own risk, are voluntarily participating in these activities, assume all risk of injury to yourself, and agree to release and discharge John Andre and Ion Som 24 Inc from any and all claims or causes of action, known or unknown, arising out of John Andre's

negligence.

Table Of Contents

Introduction

Welcome! My name is John Andre, and I am a natural bodybuilder with over 20 years of workout experience. I was first introduced to bodybuilding as a 15 year old high school student, and it has been my favorite hobby ever since. During high school, I ran on the track team for 3 seasons, and continued on to do one more year in college. I also began power lifting in 1999, and have since competed in over 20 power lifting competitions. My unique experiences with both track and field and power lifting eventually led to my interest in bodybuilding.

Although I no longer compete in track and field, I still sign up for several fun runs every year, and occasionally, I will train for a power lifting competition. I am currently considering entering into my first ever bodybuilding contest in 2015.

I hope you enjoy my workout guide. I have become a lifelong fan of bodybuilding, and I will continue to promote and support the sport as much as possible. You can follow my updated training and running advice on my blog, **www.theofficialjohnandre.com**.

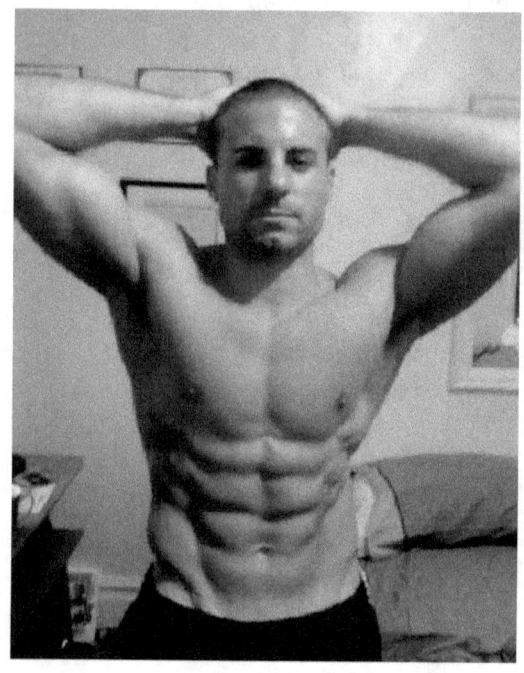

-John Andre

CHAPTER 1: INTRODUCTION TO

WORKING OUT

Working out, and especially natural bodybuilding, is one of the healthiest physical activities in the entire world. The added health benefits from exercising regularly include increases in muscle strength, stamina, and endurance. In addition, scientific studies have proven that exercise can assist in lowering a person's blood pressure, preventing heart disease, and, in my personal experience, slowing the aging process.

So who am I? My name is John Andre, and working out has been my favorite hobby since I was 15 years old. After many years of working out, I have discovered the best ways to completely burn off my extra body fat. Bodybuilding doesn't consist of just throwing shit at a wall and hoping that something sticks; it is a planned,

thought-out operation, which I have perfected through trial

and error. With this book, I wanted to weed through the

extreme amount of misinformation available on the

Internet, and help people focus on achieving actual results.

With almost 20 years of bodybuilding and workout

experience, I believe I have found the best ways to

naturally build a 6-pack.

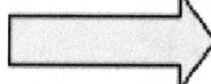 **"How Long Does It Take to Burn Off BodyFat?"**

(It takes around 5 minutes! Stand up from the couch,

perform 25 squats in your living room, and finish only half

of your dinner.)

"Working out" is a general term often used to

describe when someone is exercising, especially when they

are lifting weights. But when you begin to focus on

specific muscularity and body aesthetics, you officially

cross the line from general exercise into actual

bodybuilding.

Bodybuilding often gets a bad rap, and

unfortunately, most people associate it with steroid use

and freaky-looking bodybuilders. But the reality is, if you

are looking to gain lean muscle mass and lower your body

fat percentage, the best way to accomplish this is by

learning and applying the basic bodybuilding principles.

Bodybuilding is made up of a combination of

weight lifting, cardio, and, most importantly, diet. Many

beginning lifters make the common mistake of ignoring

their diets, but in bodybuilding, a proper diet is essential

for removing your extra body fat. Learning how to eat

properly is one of the greatest takeaways of learning some

of the bodybuilding basics, and hopefully, the good eating

habits will stick with you for the rest of your life.

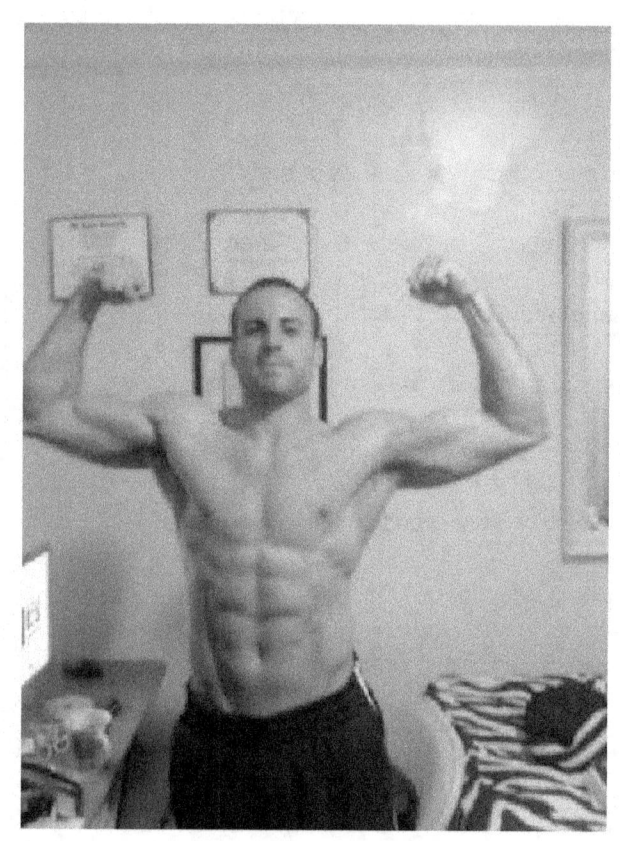

(June 29, 2012)

CHAPTER 2: YEAR-LONG PLANNING

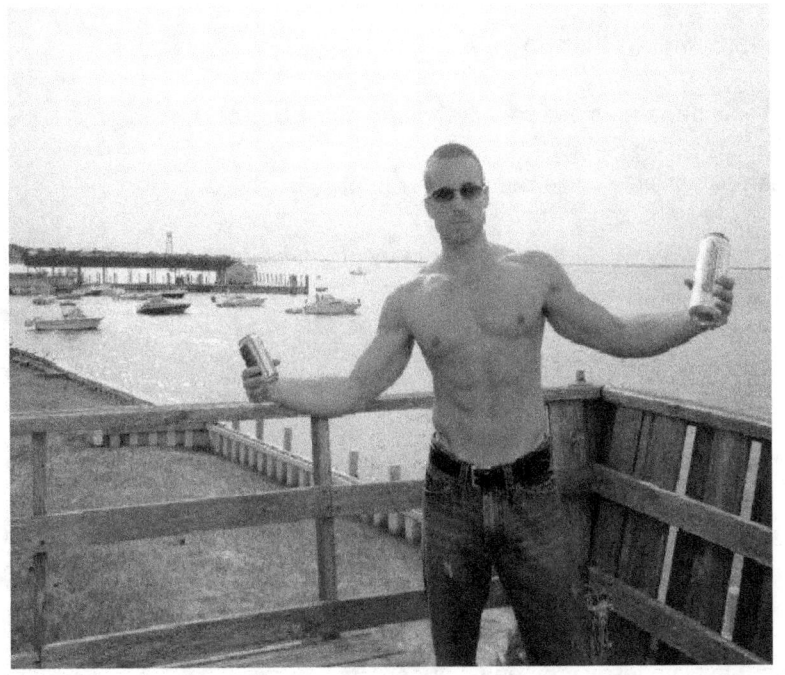

(Fire Island, Summer 2013)

At what point during the year do you want to look

your best? I personally like to plan out my training routine

almost a year ahead of time. Where I live in New York

City, it is pretty easy to plan my training around the seasons.

In the winter, I like to bulk up because it is cold and dark outside, and in the spring and summer I try to get as lean as possible while the weather improves.   Don't get me wrong, I always train year-round by lifting weights and doing cardio, but I don't always diet to the extreme level that would take my body fat percentage very low. During the winter, I will usually "allow" myself to gain some body fat, while I gradually start lifting heavier weights inside the gym. I also try to run outside year-round, but, honestly, sometimes I don't make it outside in the extreme cold.

"Bulking up" is a common term used today, and it does have some merit when done properly. Most professional bodybuilders today allow their body fat to increase in their "off-season" as a way to add-on muscle mass. When bodybuilders refer to their "off-season", they are generally speaking about the time of year when they aren't competing in any bodybuilding shows. Similar to other professional athletes who have several weeks off between seasons, professional bodybuilders also have time off between major competitions.

The reason they "bulk up" during their off-season is because it is very difficult to only put on "lean" muscle. When you gain a significant amount of body weight while lifting heavier weights, it "guarantees" that some of the mass you are adding on will be solid muscle.

The only problem I have when people start "bulking" up is that a lot of people in the gym never come back down. It isn't healthy to be overweight for an extended period of time, and I have had numerous workout partners over the years who have been diagnosed with high-blood pressure, sleep apnea, and other common illnesses associated with obesity. In the last several years, I have "allowed" myself to gain 15-25 lbs in the winter, but I always make sure I cut back down for the start of the spring and summer.

The legendary Joe Weider was known for saying, *"You need to get out of shape to get into shape."* I agree with that statement to some extent. It is impossible to diet and train at 100% intensity for the entire year, so there are going to be periods where you are training at a super-high intensity and periods when you are not. However, if you are working out consistently and eating "cleanly" all year round, you should always look pretty "good". If you are not satisfied with just looking "good", then you need to plan out a strategy to reach your full potential.

There are 2 different training plans I like to follow.

A) 8-12 week cutting schedule: This is the most

common program that most of the professional

bodybuilders utilize.   If I were training to be in peak shape

for the July 4th weekend, I would usually start this plan in

late March or early April. After several months of heavy

weight-lifting and increased calories, I start to become

very strict on my diet, and I also increase the intensity of

my cardio workouts. Similar to peeling back an onion,

when you start to increase your cardio intensity and lower

your caloric intake, your body fat will gradually start to

disappear. I am only 5'8" with a small frame, but last

year, I went from a peak body weight of 175lbs down to

155 during the summer.

There are two key components that will determine if this

method will work for you:

1) The amount of solid muscle you have built up on your frame *before* you start losing weight.

2) The amount of solid muscle you can retain *after* you lose weight.

Unfortunately, your muscles will also shrink while you cut down on body weight. The goal is to use your diet and weight lifting to preserve as much muscle mass as possible.

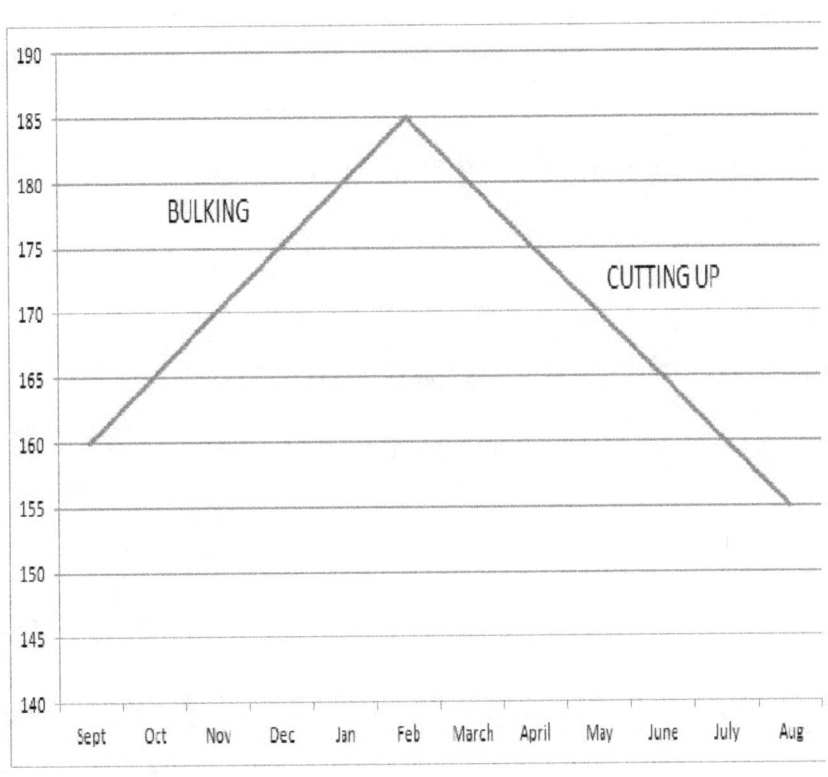

B) Waves: This is a method I personally designed, and I believe it works better for my body than the traditional 8-12 week cutting schedule. With the traditional 8-12 week cutting schedule, I always feel that I put on too much body fat during the other 40 weeks of the year.

With the "**WAVE**" system, I allow my body weight to rise

up and down multiple times within the same year. I prefer

this method because it prevents me from adding too much

extra body fat when I start bulking up. Body fat can be

really stubborn and difficult to burn off. That's why I

recommend you always eat cleanly and continue doing

cardio workouts, even during your bulk up period.

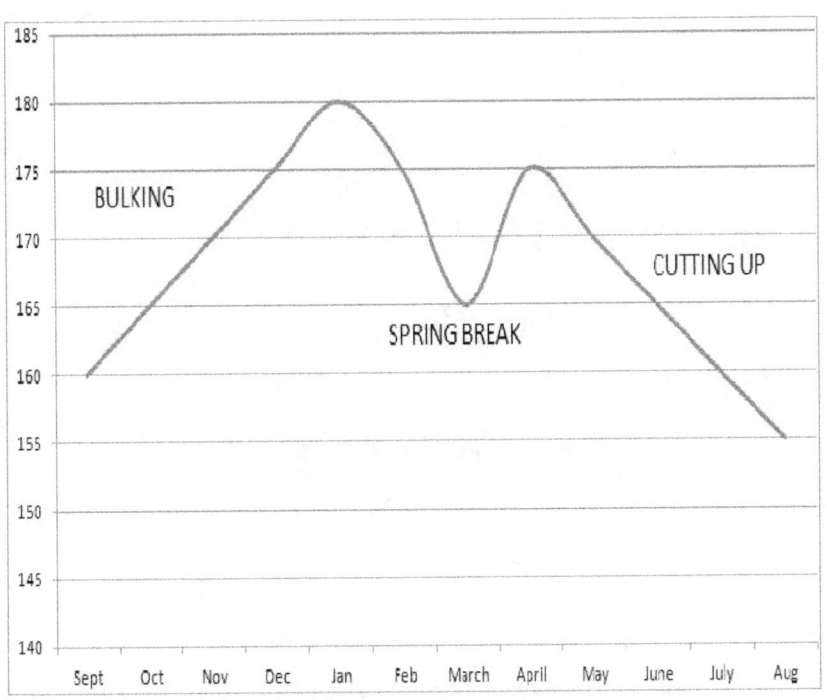

Last year, I used the "Wave" diet for a trip to

South Padre, Texas in late March. I started my year off by

bulking from September 1st until Jan 1st, but then I added

an 8-week moderate calorie-reduction diet just for the

vacation. After I returned from Texas, I started to bulk up

again until May 1st, and then I started a severe

calorie-restriction diet to officially get ready for the

summer.

For this spring break trip, I still carried some bulk,

but I cut off just enough body fat so I didn't look

overweight. In the picture below, you can see that my

6-pack was starting to come in, but it would take at least

another 10lbs of weight loss for me to get completely

ripped.

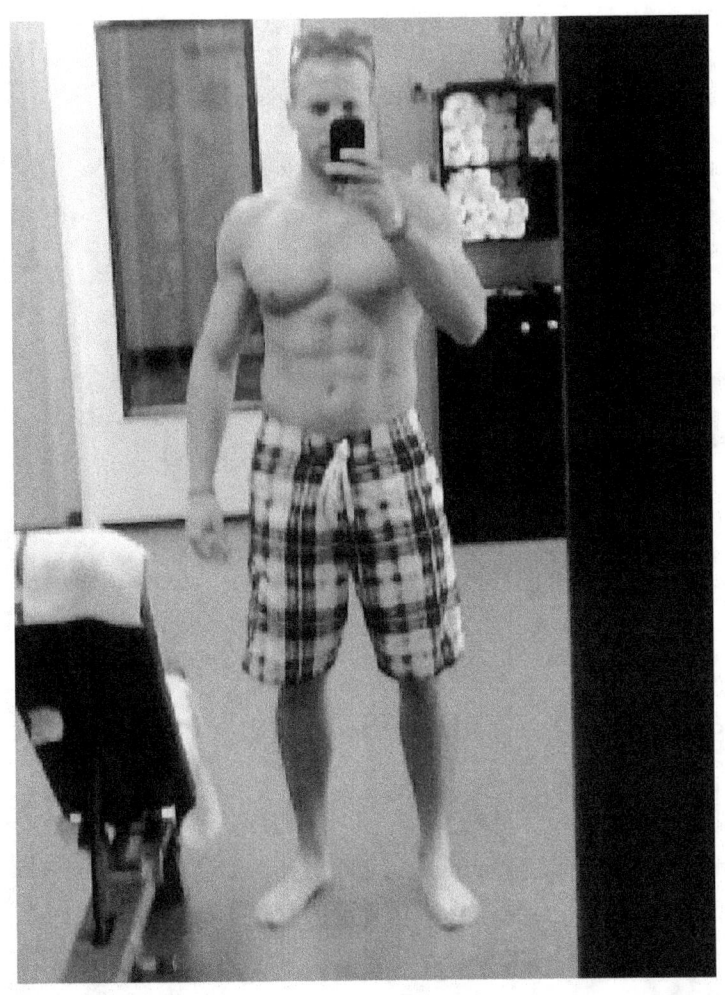

(The hotel gym in South Padre, Texas)

You can also use the "WAVE" system with your cardio workouts, which we will discuss in greater detail in chapter four.   The reason I am not including your weight training here is because your weight training routine really shouldn't change. You should always be striving to lift heavier weights, no matter how much you weigh. Of course, that doesn't mean that you can jump onto the bench press at any time of the year and break your one-rep max; you need to work "up" to it. But let me state something quite bluntly: "**lowering the weights and completing high repetitions will not give you cuts.**" You will only get "**cut**" from a combination of heavy weight lifting, cardio, and a healthy diet.

OVERWEIGHT BODY TYPES

If you are already overweight, you may want to reconsider bulking up at all. Depending on your size, you may need some extra time to burn off all of the extra body fat you have accumulated over the years. In this situation, I would avoid any bulk up cycling until your body fat returns to a normal level.

SKINNY OR UNDERWEIGHT

If you are considered "skinny" or "underweight", you should have no problem bulking up. As soon as you start to lift heavier weights and increase your caloric intake, the extra body mass should appear immediately. If you are skinny or underweight, I would also make sure that you don't go overboard with your cardio workouts. Feel free to throw in some sprints and tempo runs but avoid long-distance running at any cost. Your main goal at

this point should be to gain weight and add muscle mass.

Chapter 3: WEIGHT-LIFTING

As I stated in first chapter, bodybuilding is a

3-pillared system of weight lifting, cardio, and diet.

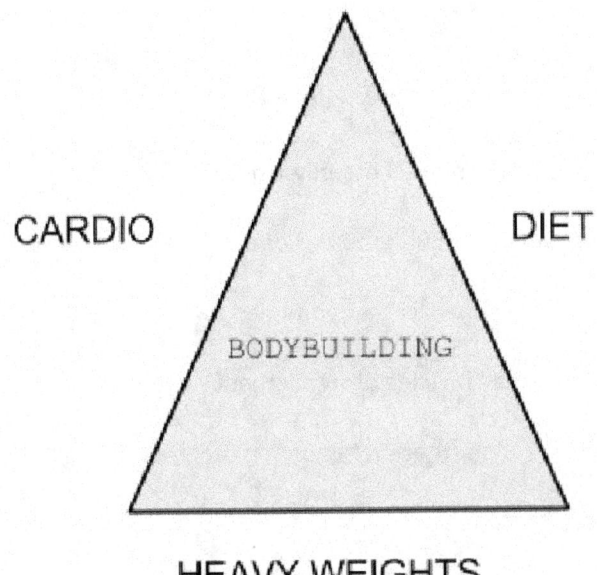

CARDIO   DIET

BODYBUILDING

HEAVY WEIGHTS

I find it difficult to give out general weight-lifting

advice because every individual person has a different

genetic makeup. What might work for one person may not

necessarily work for someone else, but through trial and error, you can discover what your body responds to the best.

Arnold Schwarzenegger recently answered some questions on reddit.com, and he mentioned that most of the famous bodybuilders at Muscle Beach trained differently from one another. The workout routine that worked the best for Arnold might not necessarily work for Ronnie Coleman, and vice versa.   But if there is one universal principle that I believe in, it is that you need to lift heavy weights to make your muscles grow. Without progressive heavy weight training, there is simply no other way to force any muscle growth.

Whether your preferable weight lifting routine consists of 10-12 reps, 4-6, or 3 sets of singles, you need to discover the perfect weight and rep scheme that will lead to the greatest amount of muscle mass on your body.

If your muscles begin to grow stronger and you can handle progressively heavier weights, then your muscles are going to grow, case closed.   The reason muscle tissue grows at all is because of the muscle tissue's reaction to the heavy stresses being placed on it. If you can fuel your muscles with the perfect amount of calories and weight lifting routine, they will grow like weeds. You just need to discover the scheme that works the best for you!   That also goes for your diet, the amount and intensity of your cardio, and even the amount of rest you need (Apparently, Schwarzenegger didn't need a lot of rest).

For the younger guys just starting out, I believe that power lifting is a great way to get started in the bodybuilding world. By starting off with power lifting routines, your body should automatically put on some solid muscle mass, and you will need that strength later on if you make the switch to bodybuilding. For example, my heaviest bench press when I was power lifting was around

350lbs, and when I started bodybuilding, that raw power

helped me to develop my chest muscles.   Because I was

accustomed to training with heavier weights, I was also a

lot stronger than most of the other guys my size. I firmly

believe that if I didn't have my power lifting background, I

would never have retained my solid upper body mass.

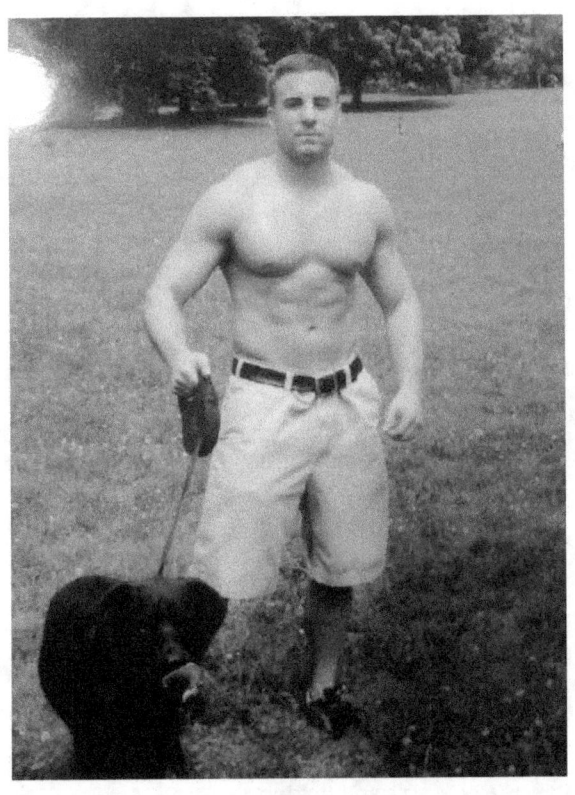

(When I was bench pressing 350 lbs)

Overall, when it comes to building mass, it is really

hard to beat some of the classic compound movements

such as bench press, squats, dead lifts, barbell curls, and

power cleans. All of these exercises are outstanding strength builders, and if you use them correctly, they will make you an overall better athlete. What exercise do I recommend to build a large chest? Bench press. What exercises do you need to build strong legs? Squats. Those are heavy, compound exercises that are very hard to replace or replicate.

One of the most common questions I receive is, "How many times a week do you work out?" I usually lift weights in the gym 4-5 times per week, and I also like to run outside for cardio at least 3 times per week. But to be honest with you, there really aren't any golden bodybuilding secrets outside of hard work. Most bodybuilding workouts are very similar. The real key is to figure out what works for YOU. For some people, 4-6 reps of heavy bench presses might make their chest muscles explode, but for other people they might need 12-15 reps with numerous sets to reach the same results.   I have had several guys tell me that the incline bench press works their chests more directly than the flat bench. Are they wrong? **They are only wrong if their chest looks like crap.** As a bodybuilder, you need to discover the exercises that work really well for you and the ones that do not.   And the only way to find out which exercises work is to experiment in the gym. Not by reading workout magazines, watching YouTube videos, or reading online forums, but by working out and figuring out your own DNA.

In conclusion, if there is one lesson I am hoping you will take away from this, it is that you need to find out what works for your body. Copying other bodybuilders is usually a waste of time. Every person has a different genetic predisposition, but in general, the basics *should* work for everyone.

THE CHEST: The chest is one of the largest upper body muscles, and fortunately, it is also one of the easiest to develop. I have found that almost anyone with normal genetics can build a large and powerful chest just by bench pressing.   The bench press is usually one of the first exercises that most beginning bodybuilders learn, and it is an outstanding exercise for building up your upper body. I have started off my weekly workouts with the bench press for the past 17 years, and I don't ever plan on changing that routine.

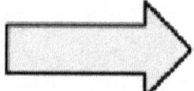 **TRAINING FOR POWER!**

When I first started bench pressing, my routine was to do 3 sets of 10 reps, and when I could complete the ten reps easily, I would increase the weight. Of course, I am assuming that you are bench pressing correctly by touching your chest and not lifting your butt off the seat. You are allowed to move your back off the bench in power lifting competitions, just as long as your traps and your tailbone are still touching the bench. In power lifting, it's called an "arch," and it can help you increase the weight you are lifting.   Most bodybuilders I know don't add too much of an arch in the gym, so I would stick with whatever feels natural. I personally arch just slightly to gain a better angle.

When it comes to chest development, my basic theory is, "If you start benching heavier weights, your chest will increase in size." It's really that simple. Every lifter should be able to eventually lift over 225lbs (two 45lb plates on each side) for multiple reps to be considered an "intermediate" lifter. If you are unable to bench press over

225lbs, you will never have a large chest unless you have really small proportions. I am only 5'8, with a small bone structure, and I have lifted 225lbs for 20 reps on several occasions.   Of course, your body weight also has to be taken into consideration. For example, a 275lb lifter should be able to lift more than a 185lb lifter, but almost all bodybuilders should eventually be able to bench over 225lbs. Over 300lbs is when you start to become an "expert" lifter, and when you can lift over 400lbs you are officially a "stud".

So, how do we increase the weight? There are a couple of routines I have used over the years. Like I stated in the beginning, if you are just starting off, you should be able to shoot up past 200lbs pretty quickly. Start with 3 sets of 10 reps, and then work your way up. When you get stuck at a plateau is when it starts to get tricky. At that point, you are going to have to change something up; either start to go heavier for fewer reps, go lighter for more reps, or I would even consider doing only 2 sets instead of 3. After a couple weeks, if you still aren't going up, you may need to increase your protein intake and gain some body weight.

When you become an intermediate lifter and you are over the 225lb plateau, I would recommend trying an old-fashioned power lifting "periodization routine". A "periodization routine" is when you start with a light weight that you can do for 12-15 reps, and then you increase the weight every week until you reach a one-rep max. For example, this is a classic periodization routine I would recommend for a bench press goal of 300lbs:

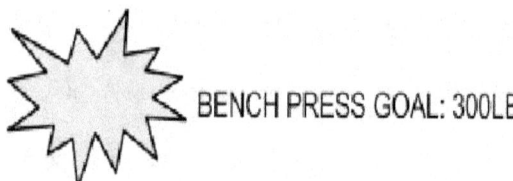 BENCH PRESS GOAL: 300LBS

WEEK 1: 205 X 15 REPS
225 X 10

WEEK 2: 225 X 10
245 X 8

WEEK 3: 245 X 8
265 X 4

WEEK 4: 265 X 6
285 X 2

WEEK 5: 285 X 4
300 X 1!

WEEK 6: MAX OUT
MAX OUT

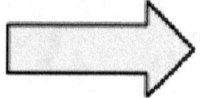 **TRAINING FOR CUTS**

Like I stated before, I firmly believe that you need to lift heavy weights to make your muscles grow, and power lifting is a great way to build a large, powerful chest. But if you want to train as a bodybuilder, you need to add some extra exercises to your routine. "Muscle confusion" is a hot topic today, and I believe in it to some extent. The human body "becomes accustomed to" or accommodates the stresses being placed on it, so after a while, the same exercises just aren't as effective. For that reason I like to mix up the exercises I use *after* the bench press. For example, I may do incline presses for 4-5 weeks immediately after bench press, but then I will switch to dips or dumbbell flys for the next 4-5 weeks. I usually only do two exercises for my chest, but occasionally, I will do three, depending on my soreness level.

Some exercises you can choose to do after bench pressing include:

39

- Dips
- Dumbbell flys
- Incline barbell or dumbbell presses
- Peck deck machine

Similar to the bench press, I would try to do 8-12 reps for each exercise, and when the sets become easy, you need to increase the weight.   I would rotate these exercises frequently to add some muscle confusion to your body. If you start to feel any extra soreness, you need to cut back.

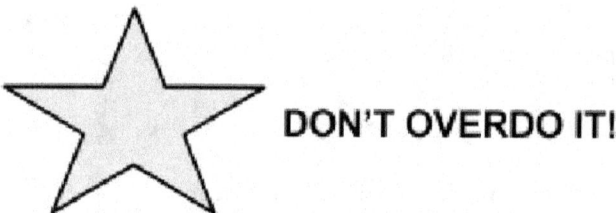 **DON'T OVERDO IT!**

The chest is a large muscle that can handle heavy poundage, but some of the supporting muscles are not as strong. Some common chest injuries include the wrists, and, most importantly, the rotator cuffs. I have injured my rotator cuffs several times from heavy chest exercises, and it is one of the most nagging bodybuilding injuries you can encounter. The rotator cuffs are involved in almost all of the upper body movements, and they are notoriously slow healers. I highly recommend that you don't go overboard with your chest exercises and if your progress starts to slow down, adding more sets can potentially make it worse.   Even though I haven't re-injured my rotator cuffs in a while, to this day, I still have to stretch out my shoulders for 20 minutes before I begin any upper body workouts.

ARMS: I like to divide the arms into 3 separate areas: the biceps, the triceps, and the forearms.

When I train my biceps, I like to stick to the very basics: heavy dumbbell curls, heavy barbell curls, and heavy preacher curls. Notice that I placed the word

"heavy" into each of those exercises. I have found that

my biceps really don't grow without using heavy weights.

When I try using a high rep routine, it makes my biceps

look strung out.

Genetics plays a large part in how your biceps will

grow. Some people have biceps that grow straight up into

peaks (the ideal for bodybuilding), while other people have

biceps that grow out long and defined. Unfortunately, my

arms are relatively long in proportion to the rest of my

body, so I need to work them with heavy weights to get

any type of "peak". Although my long arms are not ideal

for bodybuilding, they give me a strong advantage in

deadlifting, and it was actually my best lift when I

competed in power lifting competitions.

For bicep training, I prefer to mix up 2 or 3

exercises at one time, and I will structure it the same way

as I do with the bench press.　I usually start with 3 heavy

sets of a basic compound movement, such as barbell or

dumbbell curls, and then I will add 2 extra sets of another

exercise that I regularly rotate.

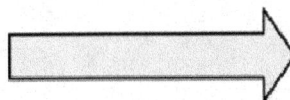

3 sets for power: Heavy barbells
or dumbbells.

+

2 sets for shape: Preacher curls,
concentration, etc

You can work out the biceps pretty hard with all

different types of drop sets, but be careful about

overworking them.　If you start to feel any type of

tearing, stop training them immediately.　I have only seen

2 people in my life tear a muscle inside the gym, and both

times, it was their biceps. If you are also training your

back hard, you may notice some extra soreness because

most of the upper back exercises incorporate the bicep

muscles.

The **triceps** are large muscles that make up

almost 2/3 of the arm. You can work out your triceps with

a variety of different barbell, dumbbell, and rope

extensions. When I'm training for power, I usually don't go

crazy with my triceps, because it weakens my bench press.

I will work out my triceps harder when I am cutting up and

sacrifice some strength to fully shape and develop the

muscle. Of course, this all depends on your genetics. If

your triceps can handle the individual attention along with

heavy chest workouts, then, by all means, blast them.

My typical routine for triceps is 3 sets with a

barbell or dumbbell, followed by 3 sets of tricep pulldowns

on a cable machine. I usually rotate between skull

crushers using barbell and dumbbell kickbacks, and on the

cable machine, I rotate between using a rope extension and a straight bar.

The **forearm** is a very basic muscle to train because there are only a limited number of exercises. Although the forearms are relatively small muscles, they can be difficult to grow. Similar to the calve muscles, the forearms are involved in so many day to day activities, it takes a lot of hard work to actually shock them into growing. I like to do 3-5 sets of basic barbell or dumbbell curls for 10-15 reps each set, and I will rotate them with 3-5 sets of reverse barbell curls. Ripped forearms look especially good when you are wearing a t-shirt, and it is also important that you strengthen your grip, so make sure you do not neglect them.

BACK: The back is a large muscle that makes up almost 60% of your upper body, and it is a very important part of your overall physique. A lot of beginning lifters will make the mistake of neglecting their back training, but a large and defined back is **mandatory** for bodybuilding.

The back can be divided into the upper and the lower. The lower back basically has 3 different exercises: good mornings, and stiff leg or regular deadlifts (if your gym doesn't allow you to drop heavy weights, then I recommend you use stiff leg deadlifts). Stiff leg deadlifts incorporate the hamstrings a lot more than regular deadlifts, but I prefer regular deadlifts because you can use heavier weights.   Deadlifting is an outstanding mass builder, and a heavy set of deadlifts to complete failure is probably the hardest exercise you can do inside a gym outside of squatting. Heavy deadlifting will add mass to your traps, legs, forearms, and even help develop your abs.

For my typical deadlifting routine, I will warm up to only one or two very hard sets of regular deadlifts or 4 or 5 sets if I am doing stiff legs. I believe the key to deadlifting is *speed*; you need to lift the weight off the ground as fast as possible if you want to get stronger. If you think you are going to slowly lift 600 or 700lbs off the ground, you are kidding yourself; you need to **EXPLODE** the weight off the ground to have any chance of lifting it. My typical deadlifting routine is as follows:

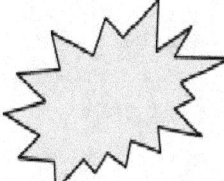 8-9 Week Sample Powerlifting Routine (Deadlift)

Week 1: 315 X 20

Week 2: 345 X 20

Week 3: 375 X15

Week 4: 405 X 12

Week 5: 435 X 10

Week 6: 465 X 7

Week 7: 495 X 4

Week 8: 525 X 2

Week 9: Max Out

Upper Back: There are a large number of exercises that you can use for the upper-back, and I recommend you completely BLAST it.   I like to start my upper-back training with a basic bodybuilding staple: chin-ups. I recommend that you work up to the point where you can do at least 10 chin-ups with just your own body weight, and then progressively add weights to your body for resistance. Most gyms usually have a belt with a chain attachment that you can hang plates from, and they are a perfect apparatus for dips and chin-ups.   I like to start with chin-ups first because they are a difficult exercise, and they become even harder when you are fatigued from other exercises.

My normal back routine starts off with 3-5 sets of chin-ups, and when I can complete 10 reps easily, I will start to add extra weight to my body.   By the time I cut down in body weight for the summer, I can usually do 10 chin-ups with a 45 lb plate attached.

After chin-ups, you can add a whole assortment of exercises including:

- Rows (barbell or dumbbell)
- T-Bar
- Seated Rows

- Machine pull downs

- Shrugs

For my typical upper back routine, I will usually do 3-5 sets of chins, 3 sets of HEAVY shrugs, 3 sets of pull downs, and 3 sets of seated rows. One added benefit of working out your back is that you should incidentally add some size to your arms. When I am training my back really hard, I notice that my biceps and forearms also start to grow larger.

Overall, the back is a large muscle and it can really take a pounding. I do both of my lower and upper back workouts during the same day, and it is usually my longest workout of the week.

SHOULDERS: The shoulders are a large and extremely important muscle group. Fortunately, the exercises needed to train them are very basic. There are really only two exercises for the shoulders: presses and raises.

Shoulder presses, with either a barbell or dumbbell, are one of the most basic bodybuilding movements.   There really isn't any substitute for heavy shoulder presses, and if you improve your strength in these lifts, your shoulders should grow larger.

I personally only do dumbbell presses now. For years I had done both barbell and dumbbell presses, but the heavy barbell presses started to aggravate my rotator cuffs. Using strictly dumbbells, I have gone up to 90 lb dumbbells for 8 reps, and 100 lbs for 2 or 3 reps. When you train with dumbbells, make sure you go all the way down, and train them hard. The shoulders are an excellent muscle to perform drop sets, and occasionally I will keep dropping the weights lower and lower until my shoulders are screaming in pain.

During my bulk up, I typically work out my

shoulders with 2 or 3 heavy sets per week after I am done

warming up. This is a sample of my recent dumbbell press

routine:

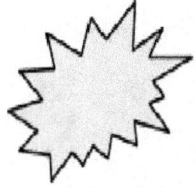 8 Week Sample Power Routine (Shoulders)

Week 1: 65's X 15, 70's X 10

Week 2: 70's X 12, 75's X 10

Week 3: 75's X 12 , 80's X 8

Week 4: 80's X 10, 85's X 6

Week 5: 85's X 8, 90's X 4

Week 6: 90's X 6, 95's X 2

Week 7: 95's X 4, 100's X 1

Week 8: Max Out

Beginning lifters should try to work their way up to

a goal of 80lb dumbbells, and then eventually up to 100

lbs.   When you start growing stronger in the shoulder presses, you will notice that your shoulders start to look like cannon balls.   If your shoulders are injury free, consider rotating between barbell and dumbbells presses, but not both at the same time. Start off with 8 weeks of barbell presses, and if your body starts to get stale, switch over to dumbbells.

The only other exercises for shoulders are raises, either to the side or the front, sitting or standing.   I prefer to do my side-raises seated, and for the front-raises, I like to stand with a 25-45 lb plate and raise it over my head with my arms locked in front of me. I rotate the type of exercises I do for raises every few weeks, and you can also do raises with the cable machine if you are getting tired of the free weights.

LEGS: I am going to share with you a little secret that I have learned about training legs. Although you might think that no one is going to see your legs during most of the year, and on the beach, you can hide them under your shorts. When you incorporate heavy leg training, it will help you A) build up your abdominals, and B) burn off a lot of body fat.

Working out your legs, especially with squats, is one of the best ways to burn off body fat and gain solid mass across your entire body. Squats are probably the first or second hardest exercise in the gym after deadlifts, and they are an exercise I recommend you learn how to perform correctly. Squatting is by far the most technical lift in the gym, and it definitely helps to have someone coach you on using proper form. Once you learn how to squat correctly, squats are one of the most absolute challenging exercises. Trust me on this, do not skip your leg workouts if you want to be in optimal shape. You will burn off body fat, strengthen your core, and add solid mass to your body.

The only real substitute for squats would be heavy leg presses, but I have tried to make the substitute in the past and I didn't see the same results. After squatting or leg presses, I will usually add 3-4 sets of leg extensions, and 3-4 sets of calves. For the calves, I like to switch between sitting calf raises, and donkey raises. To be honest, I don't go crazy with extra leg exercises because I also run outside 3 to 4 times a week and deadlift within the same week. Running outside is very taxing on your legs (especially sprinting), but if your body can handle it, then go ahead and attack it hard.

MY BASIC WEEKLY ROUTINE: This is the routine I usually follow during the year. I will often rotate my cardio workouts during the week, depending on my work schedule and other obligations. On the weekends, I occasionally like to sign up to run a race for my cardio workout and training barometer.

Monday: Chest/Forearm/Abs

Tuesday: Legs/Biceps/Cardio

Wednesday: Rest/Abs

Thursday: Back/Cardio

Friday: Shoulders/Tricep

Saturday: Cardio/Abs

Sunday: Rest

CHAPTER 4: CARDIO

I am a firm believer that you need to do some type of cardio to get ripped. Besides the added health benefits, cardio and dieting are the only ways for natural athletes like myself to burn off any body fat.   There are several different workouts you can use for your cardio, including:

SAMPLE CARDIO WORKOUTS

Tempo Runs (2-5 Miles)
Long Distance (5+)
Sprints
Sports (Tennis, Basketball, etc)
Bike Riding
Swimming

For my particular body type, I prefer tempo runs of 2-5 miles and sprinting to any type of long-distance running.   I also make it a point to always do my cardio **AFTER** the gym.   You need to be fully rested to make any progress in the gym, and cardio workouts can completely sap your weight-lifting strength. Likewise, I have never had a problem with doing cardio after I was finished lifting weights; it actually helps to stretch my body out.

Like I stated above, there are several different exercises you can use for your cardio routine, but I will only discuss the 3 main running routines: tempo runs, sprints, and long-distance.

Tempo Runs:

Tempo runs are 2-5 mile jogs at a relatively difficult pace. For my tempo runs, I like to set up concrete goals of under 6 minutes for one mile, 13 minutes for 2 miles, and 3 miles in under 20 minutes. I used to run track in college, so I wouldn't expect everyone to reach those numbers. However, try to set a minimum target of under 7:30 for one mile and 2 miles in under 16 minutes. As a rule of thumb, you should at least be able to qualify for the U.S. Army.

For my tempo runs, I like to use several predetermined courses in my neighborhood to "monitor" my progress. For example, the campus where I went to college was surrounded by a 2.8-mile oval trail, so I would run the course 4 to 5 times a week with my roommate. By the end of the semester, we were usually completing the course at least a minute or two faster, and that is how we knew we "improved." A rule of thumb to tell if you are running fast enough is that you should be able to "talk" while you are running, but you shouldn't be able to "sing". Anything less than 1 mile would be considered sprinting, and anything over 5 miles would be considered "long distance". Tempo runs are right in the middle as far as distance goes, and these runs are outstanding for burning off body fat. Tempo runs are also really good for cardio maintenance, and they are my favorite running routine during the winter.

Sprints: Sprinting has been called the **"holy grail of cardio exercises"**. When done properly, sprinting can immediately burn off your body fat, and can even increase your muscle size.   As a general precaution, if you jump straight into a sprinting routine, there is a good chance you will get injured. I recommend that you have a solid base of tempo runs before you get started on sprints. I have always found that I could perform tempo runs for several months at the time, but when I was sprinting, I would often burn out after only a dozen workouts or so. Also, make sure that you stretch out before you start a sprinting routine so you don't pull any muscles. Be especially careful about your calves and hamstrings; most sprinting injuries come from that general area.

There are several sprinting routines I recommend, such

as:

- Suicides (running back and forth between a very

  short distance)

- Hill sprints (Short sprints up a hill)

- 200 + 400 meter track intervals (one lap or half a lap

  around a standard track)

I usually warm up with a slow 1-2 mile jog before I start

sprinting, and I like to regularly mix up my routines to

prevent burn out.

Long Distance: I am not a big fan of long distance

running (5+ miles). In my personal experience, long

distance running will burn off a large percentage of your

muscle mass, weaken your joints, and destroy your

immune system. Each time I try adding long distance

running to my workout routine, my body ends up looking

terrible. With long distance running, I end up burning off

more muscle mass than I do fat, and the energy I expend

made me extremely weak in the gym. Whenever I have

increased the distances in my training, my fat burning

would suddenly drop off a cliff. I firmly believe that the

key is to focus on intensity over distance when it comes to

cardio.

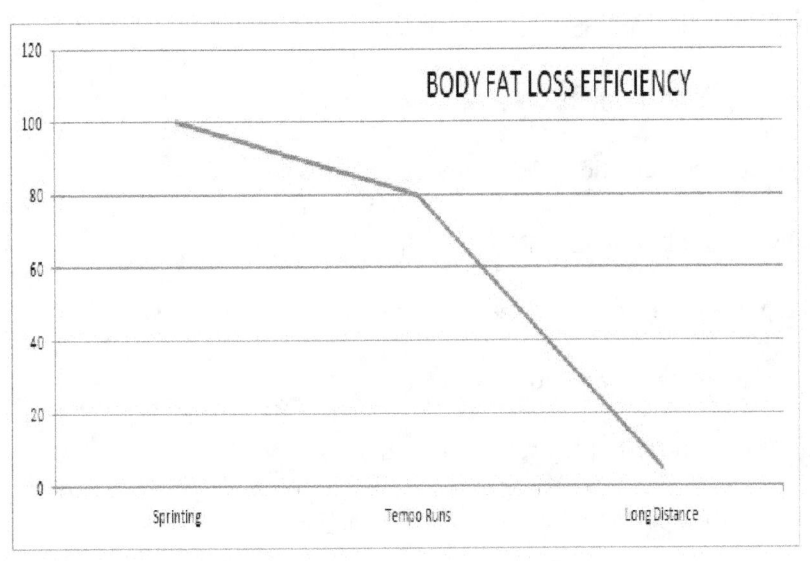

BODY FAT LOSS EFFICIENCY

Sprinting	Tempo Runs	Long Distance

Another interesting thing about running is that you don't really lose that much stamina and endurance as you grow older, but you definitely lose SPEED. All across the country, you will see plenty of middle-aged adults jogging outside, but you rarely see anyone sprinting. In today's world, there are several 70-year old men who can run a marathon in under 3 hours, but I doubt you will see any 70 year-old men dunking a basketball or playing soccer.

Stamina and endurance doesn't fade away as much as speed and muscle strength. That is why I highly recommend a combination of sprinting and tempo runs instead of long, slow, long-distance runs.   If anything, I feel like my endurance has increased in my mid-30s compared to my teens and 20s.

If you prefer to play sports instead of running, I recommend the sports that mimic the combination of sprinting and tempo runs. Tennis, basketball, soccer, and roller blading are all great alternatives to running. Sometimes when I feel burnt out from running, I start playing basketball for a couple of weeks just to mix things up.

My typical cardio schedule when I am cutting up for the summer is as follows:

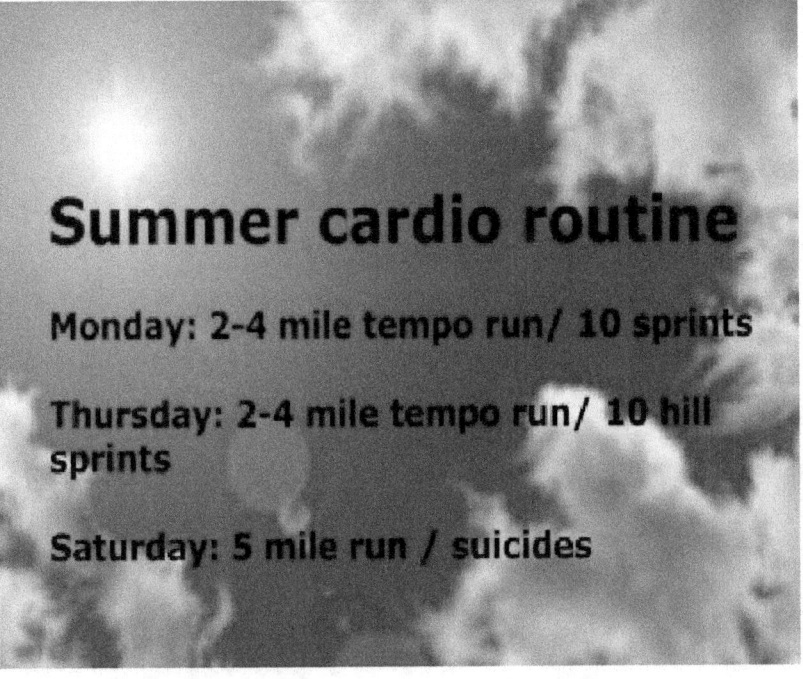

Summer cardio routine

Monday: 2-4 mile tempo run/ 10 sprints

Thursday: 2-4 mile tempo run/ 10 hill sprints

Saturday: 5 mile run / suicides

Like I stated before, I find it difficult to sprint over the course of an entire year, so I periodically take breaks to give my body a rest.   Even in the "bulking" season, though, I still like to get outside 2 or 3 times a week just to do some tempo runs. Occasionally, I will throw in some sprints if the weather permits.

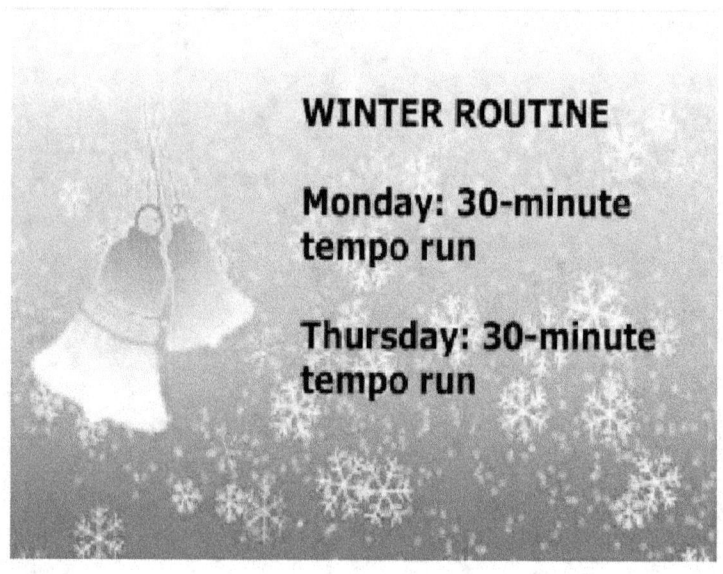

WINTER ROUTINE

Monday: 30-minute tempo run

Thursday: 30-minute tempo run

Overall, running is very addictive, but just make

sure that you don't overdo it.   A lot of beginning runners

start to get excited when they see the body fat coming off

their bodies, but then 3-mile runs turn into 10-mile runs,

10 miles turn into a half marathon, and then

half-marathons inevitably lead into marathons. And don't

forget, no one in the world has more unattractive

physiques than marathon runners.

CHAPTER#5 DIET

How important is your diet? Take a look at these before and after pictures of me.

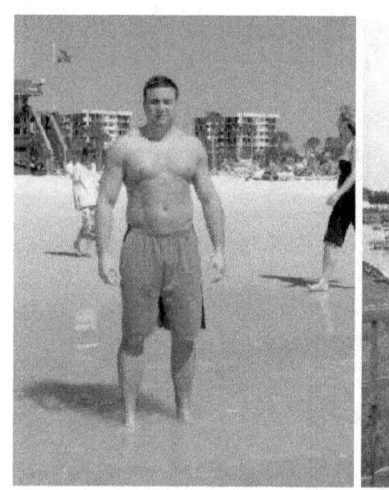 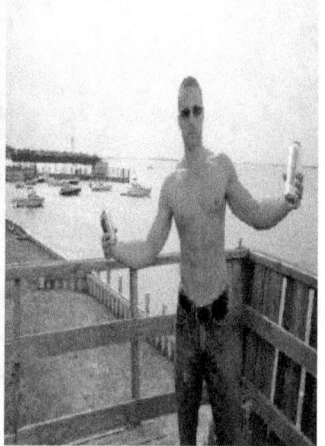

(205 lbs)   (155 lbs)

Believe it or not, I was actually using the same

exact weight lifting routine when both pictures were taken.

The only difference is that with the picture on the right, I

was using a low-calorie diet combined with 3 days a week

of outside cardio, while on the left I was only using weight lifting.   That is an example of how much of a difference your diet and cardio can make to your overall physique.

Unfortunately, the American diet is spreading across the world and it is destroying the health of many nations in its wake.   The American diet generally focuses on packing the largest amount of calories into the lowest price per unit. Factory processed goods have replaced what used to be a self-sustainable agrarian society, and the end result has been an explosive increase in obesity, heart disease, diabetes, and other self-inflicted illnesses.

Sugar is subsidized by the government, which makes it very inexpensive to use, and it is one of the most addictive chemicals known to man.   At one point in my life, I tried to completely cut out sugar from my diet, and I couldn't believe how much sugar I was consuming without even realizing it. The basic condiments like ketchup, mustard, and mayonnaise that I used for years were *packed* with sugar, and the popular sports drinks are even worse!

In some respects, you can't really blame people for the way that we eat. In the last 50 years, the United States has completely eradicated hunger. Poverty and hunger used to go hand in hand, but now the poor in this country have an obesity problem.   My grandmother used to tell me stories about how excited she was when processed goods, especially frozen goods, were first made available in her neighborhood. Before refrigeration it was very difficult to store food for long periods of time, and my family like others, became obsessed with American, brand name, consumer goods. The "Great Depression" generation was not worried as much about how their foods were being preserved or processed, they just wanted to be able to feed their families.

The good news in the United States is that more people are working out, running races, and taking various exercise classes than ever before. Let's be honest, though, most people are still overweight, and the average American is much heavier than 50 years ago.

Often you will hear a bodybuilder say, "*The Diet is everything.*" I don't want you to believe that your diet is *everything,* per se, but to be honest with you, it probably determines a large portion of your total physique. You can always "**over eat**" a hard workout. That is also another reason that I'm not a big fan of slow, long-distance cardio. You don't need to do an exorbitant amount of cardio if you learn how to eat properly.   There isn't much of a difference between burning off 500 calories during an easy run and just eating 500 calories less. Cardio will help with improvements in your cardiovascular system, but it can also have negative effects if you over do it. A good example I like to use is marathon runners. Even with the miles of training they do, they still don't have a very low body fat. I prefer the physique of an Olympic sprinter or soccer player to any type of long-distance runner.

BASIC NUTRITIONAL GUIDELINES FOR BODYBUILDERS:

Understanding proper nutrition is essential for all bodybuilders, and if you start to take your diet seriously, you will accelerate your progress. It is very important for all new trainees to understand the basic differences between proteins, carbohydrates, and fats.

PROTEIN: All bodybuilders should know about the benefits of protein for both weight training and building muscle. Increased protein intake is an absolute requirement for making maximal gains, especially when you are bulking up. The rule of thumb for protein is slightly less than 1 gram/pound of body weight, and this is plenty as long as you're getting enough calories and the sources of protein are high quality. There are a lot of good food sources of protein: meat, fish, poultry, beans and dairy, and even vegetables contain a small amount.

Protein Powders can also provide a convenient way to increase your protein intake for people who are having trouble using only natural sources. Please be careful! Most of the popular protein powders have high sugar contents, so make sure you read the label before choosing a brand. Let the mirror be your guide; if you start gaining too much body fat, then you need to cut back.

FATS: If there is one place that many bodybuilders go wrong, it is when they try to eliminate all of the fats from their diets. We do need certain types of healthy fats in our diet, but there are also others we should try to avoid. When it comes to fats, the quality is far more important than the fat quantity. As a basic rule of thumb, a fat intake of 20-25% coming from healthy sources such as vegetable oils, seeds, nuts, etc., should be consumed by all trainees.

These "healthy fats" help to provide sufficient calories without being excessive. Saturated fats from animal products (and oils like coconut and palm kernel oil) should be minimized because they are associated with health problems. Heart disease runs in my family, so I have recently tried to cut down on the amount of red meat I consume, but if your vital signs are in good order, feel free to add steak to your diet.

CARBOHYDRATES: The latest craze in the United States during the last several years has been the "low-carb" diet. Studies have shown that a high-carbohydrate diet may result in increased body fat, diabetes, and other health related problems. A high-carb diet boosts blood sugar levels, prompting the pancreas to produce more insulin to handle the excess glucose. Over extended periods, a diet high in carbohydrates can cause cells to become resistant to insulin, a major cause in type 2 or adult-onset diabetes.

Although you need to be careful about your carbohydrate intake, you still should not eliminate them completely from your diet. Many athletes tend to over-consume carbohydrates (especially highly refined ones) in lieu of healthy fats, but healthy complex carbohydrates are very important in bodybuilding. Carbohydrates are required for high-intensity training, and a lack of carbohydrates in your diet can slow down your gains in the gym.

In general, carbohydrates should make up 50-55% of a trainee's overall diet. Of that percentage, some should be starchy foods such as breads and grains, with the other portion coming from high-fiber vegetables and fruits. That ensures adequate glycogen levels for training along with adequate fiber and nutrient intake.

You should also intake a large amount of carbohydrates right after training (preferably with protein) as this has been shown to improve protein synthesis and recovery. I will usually cut down on my carbohydrates for several days in a row when I am cutting up, but then I will re-load for a day or two before going low again. During my bulk up, I am more concerned with gaining muscle size, so I will generally consume a steady amount of carbohydrates during the entire period. Like I stated above, using a low-carb diet for too long can really sap

your energy levels, so I recommend that you experiment

first to see how your body reacts.

FRUITS AND VEGETABLES: Another area where

many trainees make mistakes is by not consuming enough

fruits and vegetables.

Fruits and vegetables are crucial for proper

nutrition, and I always have at least five to seven servings

per day. Unfortunately, most fruits contain sugar, so I

recommend that you have the actual fruit instead of any

type of juice. The primary sugar in fruit is fructose, along

with water, fiber, and other nutrients. Many fruits also

contain phenols, a form of antioxidant that offers many

health benefits including protection from heart disease,

cancer, and other damaging effects of free radicals in the

body.   Overall, a limited amount of fruit is fine, and

almost all vegetables are safe for bodybuilding, especially the "greens". Most importantly, the high fiber from fruits and vegetables will keep your colon healthy and improve your nutrient assimilation.

WATER: All bodybuilders should drink a significant amount of water. At least one or two clear urinations per day should be your daily goal. Many people try to survive on just soda and coffee, but those drinks are not adequate substitutes for water. Water is important for cleansing out your system, removing sodium from your body, and helping with muscle separation. Be especially careful when you are training outside in the summer; dehydration can become a serious health problem.

GAINING WEIGHT: It amazes me how many people I meet that who have trouble gaining weight. To gain mass, you simply need to take in more calories than your body requires. Either your body will burn off the excess, or it will be deposited as tissue in your body. What type of tissue (muscle or fat) depends on how intensely you're training, how much you're eating, and the quality of the food you are eating.

If you are having trouble gaining weight, the solution is simple: start to eat more. You just need to keep adding calories until you start moving up in body weight.

BULKING UP CLEANLY: As I've grown older (34), I've found it much harder to burn off stubborn body fat as my metabolism slows down. To cut down on the amount of body fat, I have been trying to bulk up "cleaner." By bulking up "cleaner", I am attempting to increase my muscle size by only using healthy foods,

instead of just eating everything.

In the past, I would often have an extra serving of

steak, but recently I've been trying to cut down on the

amount of red meat I eat. Like I stated before, heart

disease runs in my family, and my father, who is a 3-time

marathon runner just had a major heart attack at age 67.

When it is practical, I try to bulk up by using mostly fish

and chicken. Fish can be expensive, but with the recent

rise in meat prices, fish is starting to become a practical

alternative. I've also started cooking all of my meals for

the week on Sundays, and I feel that this habit is the best

way to ensure that I don't cheat on my diet during the

work week.

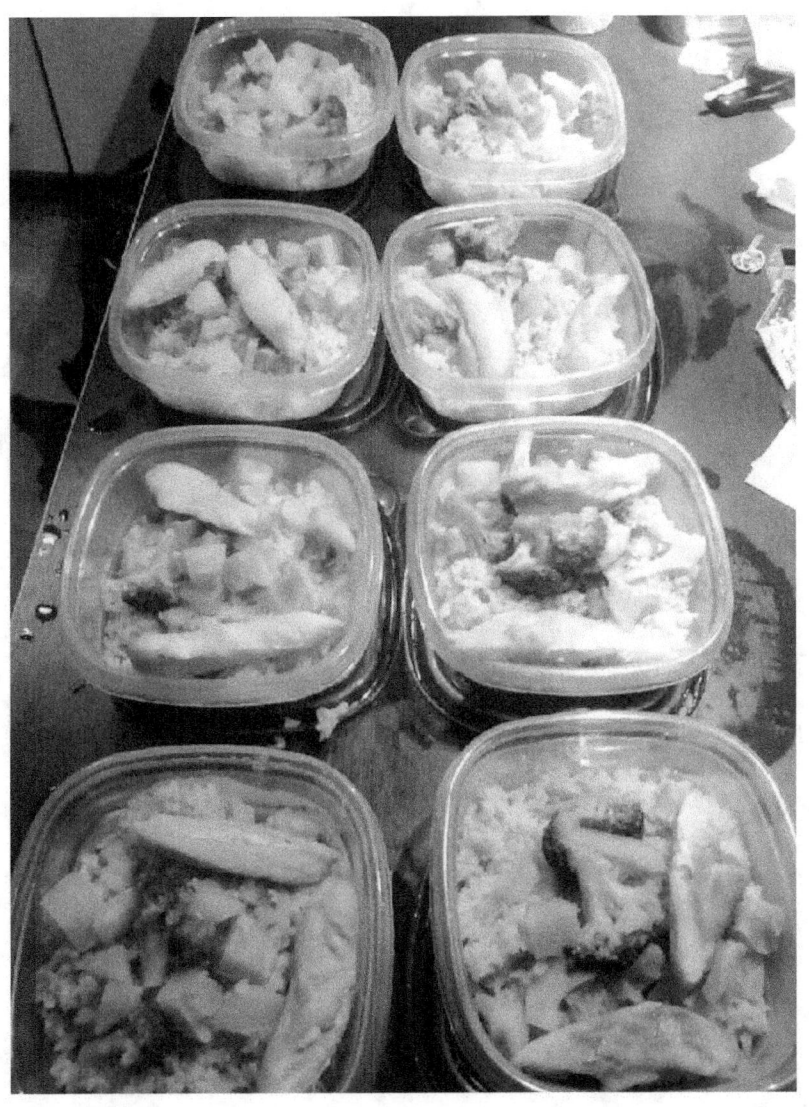

(Lunch and dinner for the week)

YOU NEED TO SEE A DIFFERENCE IN YOUR

PHYSIQUE:

Overall, when you start working out, you **need** to see a difference in your physique or you are doing something wrong. You should be either gaining weight or losing weight; maintenance is not going to work if you are trying to become a serious bodybuilder.

After bulking up for several weeks, at some point you are going to want to shed the "winter coat", and start showing off your lean muscle. When I start to shed the weight I try to stick with very clean protein sources: chicken, tuna, eggs, and steak. I also cut down on the amount of carbohydrates I take in, and when I do have them, I try to stick with low-gylcemic sources like sweet potatoes or brown rice. My usual goal is to lose 2-3lbs of body weight each month, and this is easily obtainable from eating smaller portions, using cleaner protein sources, and increasing my cardio.

Once you start cutting up, you need to stick with your diet, and over time you will start burning away all of your body fat. It may take a while, but you have to stay persistent until your body fat percentage reaches a really low level. For a lot of people, the diet is the hardest part. It takes a lot of discipline and will power, but I always find it to be pretty easy once I get into a good routine. There are a couple of tricks I recommend for when you are ready to shed the extra weight.

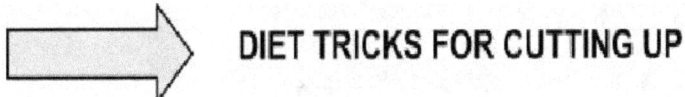 **DIET TRICKS FOR CUTTING UP**

Always feel a little bit hungry

My personal rule of thumb when I am cutting up is to always "feel a little bit hungry". When I feel the rumbling in my stomach, I know that my body is burning off the fat. I make sure that I never over-eat, and when I have that slightly uncomfortable feeling in my stomach, I know that my diet is working.

During the first couple weeks of dieting, I usually feel a little bit sick to my stomach, but after a while the pains gradually go away and my body makes the adjustments. Basically, when you start dieting, you need to calm down your "appetite". Similar to weaning off drugs or alcohol, you need to slowly "wean" off your dependency on your current caloric intake. Once you are able to control your appetite, the dieting part of your training becomes a lot more manageable.

Fasting

Another diet trick I have discovered is fasting. Fasting goes against everything modern bodybuilding stands for, but I have found it to be extremely effective in burning off fat.

The practice of fasting has been around forever, and almost every major religion has incorporated some type of fasting into its religious practices. I occasionally like to fast after I know for sure that I ate too much, or I will incorporate it with some "empty stomach" cardio on the weekends. It's hard to fast during the work week when I have other obligations, but one of my favorite weekend routines is to fast all the way up until dinnertime.

OVERALL DIET

The diet is one of the most important areas of bodybuilding, and I highly recommend that you spend a lot of your attention focused on it. My diet has evolved over time from basic trial and error. Basically, I will test different foods out and see how my body responds to them to determine if I will use it in the future. Just like everyone has different allergies and different reactions to certain medicines, people also react differently to certain food groups. The key is to try to discover whatever your body does not react well to, and try to eliminate it from your diet.

The diet is absolutely one of the most important parts of bodybuilding. If you take it seriously, you will see a tremendous improvement in your overall physique.

Chapter 6: ADVANCED TRAINING

Like it or not, your body will do everything it can to take the easy road. The human body is an adaptation machine; if you use the same training and workouts week after week, your body will eventually grow accustomed to the workload. As your body adapts to your training and becomes more efficient, you will stop making gains.

By using just the basic bodybuilding principles you can build an outstanding physique, but if you want to become a real champion, you are going to have to experiment with different routines.

Depending on your training and genetics, there are going to be certain body parts that will always look better than others. For me, my chest has always been my strong point. I need just a couple of sets on the bench press, and my chest muscles start growing immediately. There also going to be some body parts that you have trouble growing, and those are the ones you need to focus on. My weaknesses, for sure, are my calves and my upper back. I am constantly experimenting with different exercise routines to try to make improvements.

I am also a firm believer that you need to find out what works best for you. Reading information on bodybuilding is almost useless, because there is no real substitute for experience. While your training partner might need only two or three sets to build up huge biceps, you may find that your biceps need 15 to 20 sets to have the same results. It is really up to you to discover how your body reacts to different training methods.

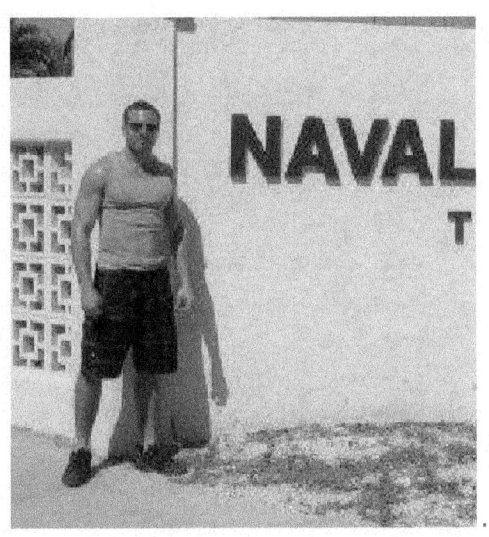

(After several weeks of heavy biceps)

These are some advanced routines that I use:

Stripping method: After a quick warm-up, I will perform an exercise that I can lift for 5 reps. Immediately after that set, I will strip some of the weights off the bar and do another 5-8 reps. Sometimes I will only strip it down for one extra set and other times, I will keep going lower and lower until I am down to just the bar. This works really well with muscles you can destroy, like the biceps and calves.

The 1-10 method: After warming up, try to do a one-rep max set. After you perform that one rep, take some weight off so you can perform two reps. Continue dropping just enough weight to add one more rep until you get up to 10 reps on the last set.

Running the rack: This is an exercise that works really well with the biceps and shoulders. I will grab a set of dumbbells I can only lift for about 6 to 8 reps. Once I complete the first set, I will drop the dumbbells and grab another pair that are 5 pounds lighter. After the second set, I will keep going lower and lower until I complete the entire rack of dumbbells.

German Volume Training: The German Volume training is when you use an extreme number of sets to train each body part. I have used this method in the past and it works really well, but make sure that you don't overwork yourself. The high-volume system works really well after you have already built up a significant amount of mass on your body. I wouldn't use this system to bulk up, but it works really well for an 8-10 week cut up.

Using this system, I will do 12-15 sets of chest in the 8-12 rep range, and for my biceps, I will even go as high as 20-25 sets. Of course, you won't be able to lift as heavy when you are doing so many sets, but it is a great way to really define your muscles.

Chapter 7: ACCOUNTABILITY

All bodybuilders need to consistently progress in their training in to see any results. Professional athletes today are still competing in bodybuilding, power lifting, and mixed-martial arts competitions up until their mid-40s. Until you reach a solid middle age, you should always be striving for increased strength and speed. Your genetics and training intensity will determine at what age you peak, but generally you should still be pretty strong into your late 40s and early 50s.

So, how do we test accountability?

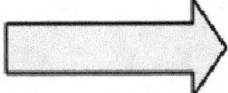 *How much can you lift, how fast can you run, and what do you look like?*

There are several straightforward tests you can use to hold yourself accountable. For example, if your max bench press is now 255lbs and last summer it was only 235lbs, that is an obvious improvement. If you are bench pressing the same amount as last year but you were able to shed off 5-6lbs of body fat, that can also be considered an improvement.

I like to use the following indicators to determine if I am making improvements:

- Bench press max

- Bench press for 10 reps

- Shoulder dumbbell max

- Shoulder dumbbell 10 reps

- Dead lift max (or heavy 2 or 4's)

- Chin-ups, non-weighted

- Chin-ups, weighted

- Squats (6-8 range)

- One-mile running time

- 3-mile running time

When you set concrete goals and hold yourself accountable, it becomes much easier to track your progress from year to year. When you start to get cut up for the summer knowing that you are **A) stronger** and **B) faster** than you were last year, then the rest of the work is all pertaining to your diet.

The majority of people you will see in the gym are just there for maintenance. They have built up a solid base of muscle, and they are only looking to maintain and stay in shape. Even if you look at the top professional bodybuilders, it is hard for them to make significant

progress year after year. The only way to make any

changes is by getting stronger, being faster, tightening up

your diet, and increasing your efforts inside the gym. Try

to hold yourself accountable, and you may be able to

continually make progress with your physique.

Chapter 8: ABS

I decided to add a separate chapter on abs

because it is a very important body part in bodybuilding.

Let's face it, every new bodybuilder has dreams of building

ripped abs, but few will ever achieve it. In bodybuilding,

there is no other body part that has historically

represented a more classic physique than a pair of chiseled

abdominal muscles. The ancient Greeks and Romans

highly respected a ripped midsection, and you can see it

clearly in their sculptures and paintings. In my opinion,

the greatest bodybuilder in history is still standing in

Florence, Italy: Michelangelo's "David".

If you were to ask a random guy or girl on the

street to show you their muscles, usually the first thing

they will do is flex their biceps. But the real truth is that almost anyone in the gym could easily build up a decent

pair of biceps, but a true bodybuilder needs to have a fully

defined set of abdominal muscles.

I am going to be completely honest with you,

achieving ripped abs is not very easy. It takes a hard,

consistent combination of cardio, diet, and weight- lifting.

It is not a coincidence that the years where I had my most

defined abs were also the years that I was in my best

overall shape. You can't really fake yourself into getting

ripped abs, and even the guys who use steroids often end

up with weird looking midsections.

The biggest mistake I see beginning lifters make is

that they add extra abdominal exercises instead of

focusing on lowering their overall body fat percentage.

Let's say, for example, that you were going to train the

famous wrestler "Andre the Giant" to get a ripped 6-pack.

Would it help him to start doing 200 crunches every night?

Of course not. You might see his waist area shrink slightly, but his abdominals would never pop out unless he lost over 300lbs. No matter how strong you are, **if you cannot remove the body fat from your body, you will never see your abdominals!**

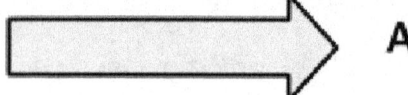 **Abdominal Training!**

Basically, there are two trains of thought when it comes to training the abdominals. The old-school bodybuilders recommend that you train your abs every day with high repetitions, while most of today's modern bodybuilders recommend that you only train them once or twice a week.

To be honest with you, after years of training, I find that my diet and cardio workouts are more important than any of the abdominal-specific exercises. The exercises that helped me the most weren't even the sit ups and crunches, per se, but the heavy squats, dead lifts, barbell shrugs, and overhead lifts. It isn't very apparent when you are bulking up, but those heavy compound movements will really help to build up and strengthen your core.

Once you start to burn off your body fat using your diet and cardio, the only thing left over is going to be your cube-shaped abs. When I say that you can't fake abdominal training, I mean it. If you were too lazy during the winter to do heavy squats and dead lifts, you will notice it in the summer when your abs aren't popping out. And if you aren't strict with your diet and cardio, you can simply forget about getting your body fat low enough.

Although I recommend the heavy compound movements, there are numerous abdominal-specific exercises you can use in your training, including:

- Crunches
- Situps
- Side twists
- Bicycle kicks
- Roman chair
- Planking
- Hanging leg raises
- Hanging knee raises
- Oblique crunches
- Scissor kicks

It is really up to you to plan out an abdominal-training routine you can follow, but, if you work hard, eat right, and train your body correctly, your abdominals should end up looking like this.

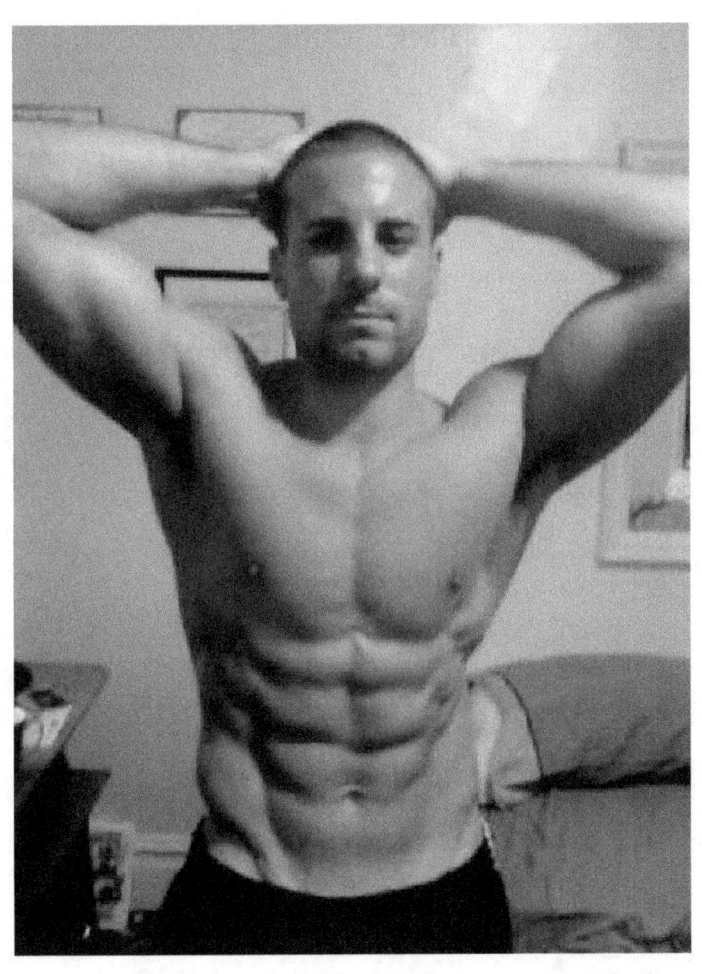

(John Andre, June 2013)

Chapter 9: FUTURE GAME PLAN

Now that we have reviewed the different workouts, along with the keys to implementing a proper diet, all we need is a well thought-out game plan.   I like to use September 1st as my starting point because it traditionally represents the end of the beach season in New York City. As the year progresses, I will periodically change my training in tune with the changes in the seasons.   This includes my weight lifting goals, diet, and the amount of cardio. But overall, I still believe it is important to incorporate all of your training into a long-term plan.

LABOR DAY TO THANKSGIVING: LEAN GAINS

The fall is my favorite time of year to run outside, and since the weather is still nice, I recommend a period of "lean-gains". By "lean-gains" I mean that I will *slowly* gain body weight while progressively lifting heavier weights in the gym. I will usually gain on average about 10lbs between Labor Day and Thanksgiving, for an average of 2.5 lbs per month. That is a safe amount of weight for me to put on without adding too much body fat.

During this time of year, I will usually lift weights 4 times per week in the gym, and I will also do tempo runs 3-4 times a week outside until it starts getting too cold.

THANKSGIVING TO ST. PATRICK'S DAY

This is the time of the year where it obviously gets very cold in N.Y.C, and there will undoubtedly be some days where it is just impossible to run outside. There are several indoor running tracks in NYC that I occasionally

use, but this is the time of year where I will do the bulk of

my heavy weight lifting in the gym. During this period, I

will gain another 10lbs of body weight and try to set new

highs in most of my compound lifts.

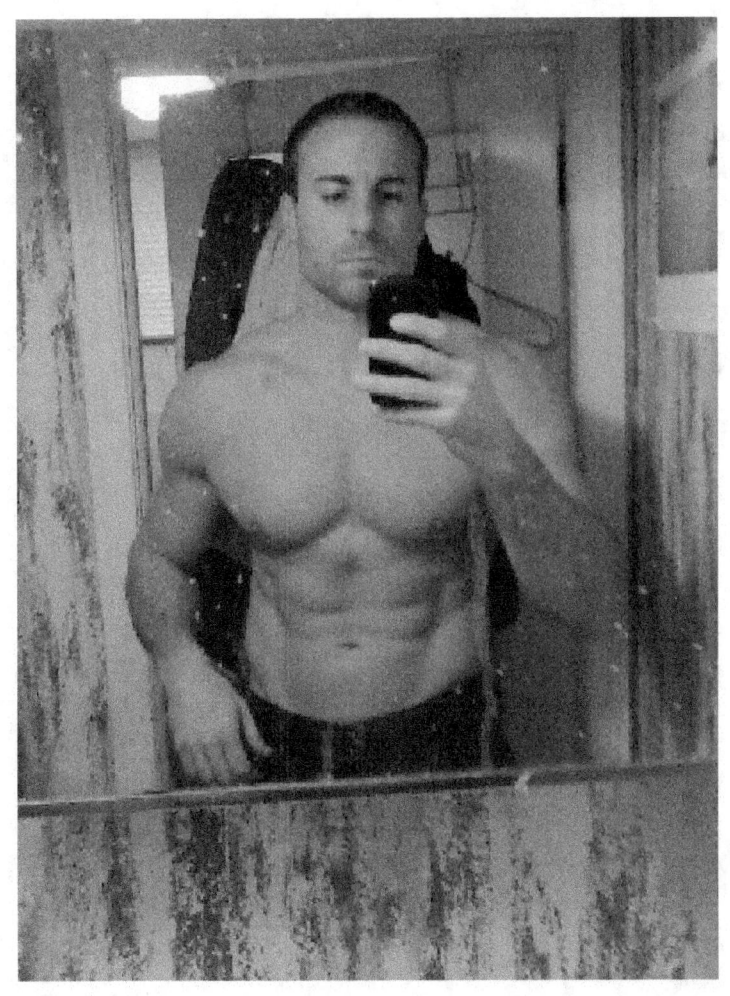

(March 1, 2014)

After St. Patrick's Day, I will slowly start to cut
down on my caloric intake, and I will also start to run
outside more as the weather improves. At this point, I will
start losing at least 2-4 lbs per month, and usually by
Memorial Day, my abs will finally start to pop out.

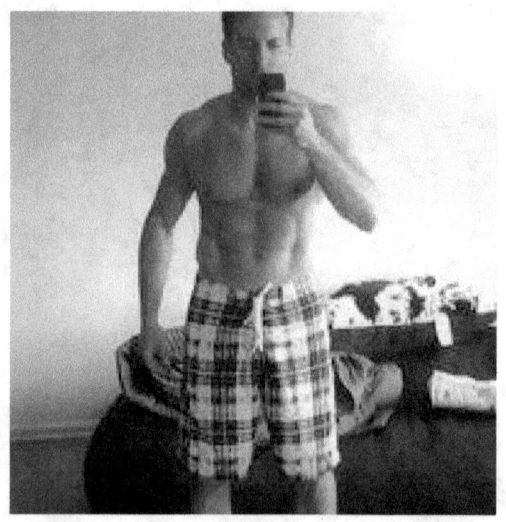

(Memorial Day Weekend 2014)

SUMMER TRAINING

After Memorial Day weekend, I will get super-strict on my diet, and I will lose the remaining 5-10 lbs of body weight until I get shredded. At this point, I will be at the lightest body weight of the entire year, and I am usually running my fastest times of the year outside. Unfortunately, I will also be at my weakest, and at this point I am usually using 10-15% lighter weights at the gym. This is the time of the year that you should look your leanest and most defined.

Chapter 10: Conclusion

If you can incorporate my training programs along with a proper diet and cardio routine, I can almost guarantee that you will see improvements in your physique.   Bodybuilding is one of the greatest hobbies in the world, and anyone who is willing to put in the time and effort can improve their physique, gain strength, and burn off most of their extra body fat. Working out has been my favorite hobby ever since I first touched the weights at age 15, and I haven't stopped yet, even into my mid-30s. I plan on lifting weights until the very end, and keeping myself in the best shape possible.

If there is any final advice I can leave you with, it is to "**do the work**".   Forget about researching online or going crazy over supplements, just get yourself to the gym, make improvements to your diet, and enjoy the

journey.

Good luck!

-John Andre

www.ingramcontent.com/pod-product-compliance
Lightning Source LLC
Chambersburg PA
CBHW062012280526
45787CB00005B/2071